A DEFINITIVE GUIDE TO KETTLE BELL TRAINING AND FAT LOSS

Disclaimer

You are viewing an **UNOFFICIAL MODEL** of the context from the book **"The Ultimate Kettlebell Training and Fat Loss Book"**

The contents of this model are not poised to replace the original book. It is meant as a complement to enhance the reader's understanding.

Once again, this complimentary guide intends to encourage the reader to get the original book to further their comprehension and understanding.

in whole or in part without the publisher's or creator's

permission.

TABLE OF CONTENTS

Will you finally say, "Enough Is Enough" at this point?

I'm prepared to embark on a path to a healthier version of myself; I won't offer any more justifications; and I'm going to effect change by losing some of those extra pounds.

Absolutely not!

If so, get ready to...

The infomercials I watch on Saturday morning and at night simply astound me. They advertise these tools and gimmicks that guarantee quick weight loss. How many of us have seen those "ab gadgets" where you rock back and forth while sitting and the fat just melts away?

Have you read the screen's bottom-most, extremely small print? In essence, it tells you that in order for it to work, you must follow some kind of diet.

Today, it is simple to fall prey to promises of quick weight loss made by some diet plans, "magic diet pills," and other "miracle weight loss diets." But in all honesty, it is a bunch of nonsense.

Before you choose your course of action, there are a few fundamental truths you should be aware of.

First of all, be aware that there is **NO** magic cure for weight loss.

While following a very strict diet or another popular fad diet can result in significant weight loss, the main drawback is that these diets are not long-term sustainable.

In addition to the obvious harm to your health, I've come to understand that the word "diet" makes me think of limitations. One definition of diet, according to the dictionary, is "a regimen of eating and drinking in moderation in order to reduce one's weight." Diets not working is not a surprise.

According to studies, the majority of overweight people who start a crash diet quickly gain back the weight they lost. When this happens, their health is significantly worse than it was when they were initially overweight.

To be honest, losing weight hasn't changed much since humans first started walking on two legs. What has changed is how weight loss tips are marketed. You must ultimately have a negative energy balance.

How do you achieve a balance of negative energy? You can first cut back on how much food you consume daily. The second option is to step up the difficulty of your workouts.

Finally, you can combine the first two strategies. I'm done now.

Having said that, this book's focus is on tried-and-true nutritional and exercise advice because there is no such thing as a miracle.

This book aims to cut through the Internet-wide BS and assist you in making the lifestyle changes necessary to reach the weight that you have determined is best for you.

CHAPTER ONE

Why Am I Getting Fat?

It sure is challenging to maintain an active lifestyle and consume a healthy, balanced diet given the pace of our modern lives, the advancement of technology, and the conveniences of fast food. But if you know how to do it, it can be done, even with a busy lifestyle.

In this first chapter of the book, we'll examine:

- Why maintaining a schedule actually aids in weight loss;
- the primary causes of weight gain;
- the people we should consult when we decide we are ready to lose the weight.
- Along with many other topics, learning about weight loss secrets will help you figure out how to finally lose the weight and keep it off permanently.

The Principal Reasons for Weight Gain

i. **We consume more calories each day than our bodies require, and the extra is then stored as fat**: We all understand this, so why are 63% of Americans overweight or obese? The portions we consume today are enormous, as you can see.

We are in a positive energy balance when we eat more than we burn. Essentially, we store the extra as fat. If we were cavemen and knew we wouldn't eat for seven days, this might be a good thing, but for those of us who live in western society, this isn't the case.

ii. **You don't get enough sleep**: It may be time to take care of any sleep problems you may have if you are dieting and exercising but are still not losing weight. In the Canadian Medical Association Journal, two Canadian obesity experts note that there is growing evidence pointing to a connection between sleep and weight loss. In fact, the study discovered that those who stay up later eat 400–500 more calories!

iii. **Your metabolism**: After the age of 25, we begin to lose 10% of our metabolic rate every ten years. If you follow the instructions in this book for kettlebell training, you can stop this from happening. In other words, when we have more lean muscle, our metabolic rate rises because our bodies need to build more muscle to repair the muscle from the workout. We gain weight when we are sedentary because this doesn't happen.

iv. **Your eating habits are subpar**: People in the West are now 30 pounds heavier than they were 100 years ago, according to my research for this book. They consumed more fat, which is even more intriguing! You see, foods high in sugars, starches, and almost anything made with flour are making us an obese society. Fast Food Facts reports that the fast food industry alone spent 4.2 billion dollars on advertising in 2009! We are fat for a reason. A meal planner has been found by many people to be helpful in pointing them in the right direction.

v. **Larger portion sizes**: This is common knowledge. Simply put, most people eat too much. This meal planner can help you understand what a portion should look like, as was previously mentioned.

vi. **Exercise or the lack thereof**: The western society is being destroyed by this. Today's children are the first generation to have a shorter life expectancy than their parents, according to designedtomove.org. The human body is built for movement. To reach and maintain a healthy weight, regular exercise is crucial. What you eat, how you eat, and how much you eat are also important factors.

vii. **Control your intake**. Use your hand to measure instead of weighing or measuring as a simple rule of thumb in this situation. Men need two portions of protein, while women only need one. Your palm would fit inside of a portion.

Both men and women should choose a portion of carbohydrates that is the size of your fist.

Protein that is the same size as your palm should be consumed by men. The majority of people frequently underestimate how much they are eating due to this factor. Generally, you should only eat a portion of food the size of your fist at a time because that is also the size of your stomach.

When you are 80% full, stop eating. This is a method that I use 90% of the time, and it will undoubtedly help you eat less. Consider portion control in this situation; there is no better way to manage what you put in your mouth than by eating less at each meal. If you do this for a year, you will lose a lot of weight.

Try eating more slowly and avoid eating while driving, standing, or moving. You should only consume food at a table. You should eat slowly because your brain receives a signal when you are full.

When you eat quickly, your brain does not receive the signal, leading you to overeat because you do not feel "full." I know you're busy, but if you substitute a healthy meal for one when you're busy, you might still be able to maintain a healthy weight.

Of course, monitoring your intake of fatty and sugary foods is another important step. To stay balanced, we all need nutrients, including healthy fats, but consuming a lot of junk food and sugary beverages will significantly contribute to our weight gain. Processed foods are typically low in nutrients, if they contain any at all, and high in unhealthy fats, salt, and sugar.

People frequently blame their busy schedules for their weight gain. To avoid falling into any traps that will force you to make poor nutrition decisions, you must really plan ahead in this situation.

You can plan your meals for the week and get a shopping list for all the ingredients you'll need with a meal planner.

Breakfast can be challenging to fit in, so to avoid making a bad decision or going without food altogether, I suggest using a meal replacement.

Do I Need to Start A Diet?

The quick response is "absolutely not" They are not long-term solutions. It's difficult to avoid falling for the hype when the newest "diet fad" is heavily marketed, as we've already discussed. Think about a lifestyle change instead of a diet because this will create long-term healthy eating and exercise habits as opposed to a quick fix diet.

Do you enjoy skipping entire food groups like carbohydrates or chugging down weight-loss drinks that just don't taste very good or fill you up?

Most people seem to begin a diet around significant life events, such as marriage, high school or family reunions, or the big one—New Year's resolutions.

If reaching a healthy weight is your only objective, I would advise you to do your research. At least you will be aware of how to keep the weight off in the long run once you have reached your short-term objective.

You must have a reason for making any kind of change to your regular daily activities before you start. These would be regarded as objectives or goals.

Goals are crucial because without them, you'll give up when things get tough. Perhaps you recently went from a size 40 to a size 42 in pants, and you're sick of being big. Maybe your doctor warned you that if you don't lose 50 pounds, a heart attack is a real possibility.

Your objectives must be sincere. Writing them down allows you to display them somewhere and be reminded of them daily. The acronym S.M.A.R.T. is the formula I prefer to use.

Specific: Starting out with only a vague idea of where you're going will guarantee failure. You wouldn't just drive to get to a particular location in New York City if you were planning to drive there, would you?

On the other hand, you would have specific instructions before leaving to make sure you arrived at your intended location. The same goes for statements like, "I want to get in better shape," which are too general to be taken seriously.

It has no force behind it, and you won't even be able to tell if you've succeeded. How so? Technically, you would be in better shape now than when you started if you just lost one pound!

Get specific and determine what you really want because it is obvious that this is probably not what you had in mind.

Consider setting a goal like, "By the end of this year, I want to lose 35 pounds and fit into the same pants I wore in college." See the distinction? If you use specifics like these, you will now be able to determine when you arrive at your destination.

Measurable: This complements the idea of keeping your goal measurable, which goes hand in hand with being specific in your statement. Why does this matter?

Make sure your statement provides a clear response to the question "how much" The answer, using the same example as above, would be 35 pounds.

To keep you on track, you can go even further with this. Create smaller milestones that you would like to reach along the way rather than just listing your overall objective.

You might say, "I want to lose 35 pounds, which means I need to lose at least 3 pounds each month for a year."

This gives you a fantastic way to monitor your development, which will keep you inspired. After all, a journey of a thousand miles begins with a single step, according to an ancient Chinese proverb. In a similar vein, it's impossible to lose 35 pounds all at once, but you can do it this week!

Attainable: It goes without saying that you must keep your objective within the bounds of reason for this one. Expecting to run on the treadmill once and lose 20 pounds in a day is unrealistic. Instead, you need to divide your objective into manageable chunks that are aggressive enough to keep you working hard but also feasible.

If not, you might give up after a few weeks of falling short of your goals. It would be better to start with a lower goal and increase it as you consistently surpass it each week.

Realistic: Realistic objectives are by definition attainable objectives, but there is a fine line separating the two. You might not be able or willing to reach a particular benchmark, even though it might be possible to do so.

For instance, while reducing your body fat to 7 percent may be theoretically physically feasible, it might not be practical. Your objective should be to get in reasonable shape if you are starting out as a couch potato or 100 pounds overweight. Trying to improve your fitness from where you are now to that of a triathlete isn't really realistic, and you risk setting yourself up for disappointment in the future.

The mere fact that something is feasible (achievable) does not guarantee that you will succeed (realistic). So, try to keep your objective in the middle, and everything should work out for you!

I want to reduce my body fat percentage from 22 to 14 percent over the course of seven months.

However, keep in mind that a difficult task might be made simpler because it will keep you motivated. Setting the bar too low may cause you to become disinterested. Only you can decide where the ideal balance lies, and if you feel like you need a little extra motivation in the middle, you can always raise your goals!

Time Determined: You've probably noticed that each example includes a particular time period. This is crucial because without it, you won't be able to make on-the-go plans.

You would only need to lose 2 pounds a month if you gave yourself two years to lose 50 pounds. You will need to double that amount, though, if your goal is to lose weight in just one year.

Therefore, a crucial component of your goal is your deadline, which needs to be very detailed.

Next, what? Now that you have a specific objective in mind that you have worked hard to make compelling, congratulations! What's the next move, and how can you make the most of this? You need to constantly remind yourself of this goal by posting it somewhere you will see it every day, as was already mentioned. This will serve as a reminder of your goals and may also aid in the formation of new routines. It only takes 21 days to establish a new routine or habit, so after three weeks of healthy eating and exercise, life will be much simpler.

However, if you've battled your weight for a long time, your eating habits and sedentary lifestyle may be deeply ingrained in you. To break out of this rut, you might need to be aggressive and try something a little crazy!

Is a negative medical report what finally motivates you to lose weight? Then display your medical records, the results of any blood tests, or simply a reminder of your poor state of health next to your stated objective.

Why on earth would you engage in such a morbid activity? You see, if you're like most people, you'll want to quickly forget about this worrying development. This is only natural because you don't want to think about uncomfortable things all the time.

But it's crucial that you do so because it might inspire you like nothing else in your life. It will become clearer to you that you cannot afford to waste this time when you see the test results or your doctor's note every morning.

Alternatively, you might have a more uplifting reason, such as fitting into a smaller dress size for a forthcoming event. Why not post a picture of the contested dress or the actual dress itself?

It may sound a little out of the ordinary, but seeing your goal right in front of you every day will make it simpler for you to say no to the donuts at work.

The image of that dress will be still in your mind when you're tempted to abandon your diet or skip your workout. Although it may seem straightforward, this actually works! Why not give it a try since you might start getting results that you have never seen before?

Get Support: You might think that you are done at this point since you have created a SMART goal and placed it in a prominent location where you will see it every day. Although this is a fantastic beginning, you still need one more thing to be successful!

You see, the reason why most people fail is that they don't set up a support system to get them through the really difficult times. These will unavoidably arise, and somewhere along your personal weight loss journey, you will feel like giving up.

It could be as simple as having a difficult day at work, soreness from your most recent workout, or depression making you want to eat an entire chocolate cake! Whatever the situation, there will be a time when you require support to get you through a difficult period.

Who should you contact to form your own support group? It should go without saying that you need a supportive partner in your weight loss efforts. Since they probably see you every day, it would be ideal if you could enlist the aid of your spouse.

Additionally, you probably share at least one meal each day with them, allowing them to observe your eating habits as well. Unfortunately, your spouse might not be open to change and even be hostile to your weight-loss plan. They might also be unhealthy, but they aren't willing to change, so they will only be a bad influence. If so, you will need additional support from other friends or family members to make up for the support you aren't getting at home.

In fact, it is best to ask a friend who is already physically fit for assistance because they are aware of what it takes to keep the weight off. Additionally, they won't be tempted to skip workouts or consume unhealthy foods, so they won't give in if you beg them to.

If you don't know anyone like this, look for a friend with whom you can get in shape so that you can work together to shed the pounds. As you can't skip your workout if you have a meeting at the gym, this can be a strong motivator. You will have an additional incentive to maintain your diet since you will be required to tell them what you have been eating.

Free Personal Training: You can benefit from my experience in addition to having a friend or spouse as a source of support. There, you can see my meal plans and the exercises I choose to do. This is similar to having a personal trainer, but without having to spend any money. Additionally, keep in mind that you can get in touch with me if you have any questions; I'm here to make sure you are successful in losing the weight.

Combining it All: You now understand how to create a fantastic goal that will keep you highly motivated. Keep your goals specific, measurable, reachable, realistic, and time-bound!

You will be able to accurately navigate and determine when you have arrived at your destination if all of these conditions are met. Then, just glance at it once a day or more to keep your new objective fresh. The next step is to enlist the assistance of your partner or a close friend to help you stay on course whenever you are tempted to stray. You will be in a good position to achieve your weight loss goals if all of these factors come into play.

How Diets Work

Losing weight is simple; Simply consume fewer calories each day than your body needs to function to lose weight.

It goes without saying that we eat because it is necessary for our bodies to function. We will put on weight if we eat more than we need. Consider this: an increase in daily caloric intake of just 300 calories could result in a 20-pound weight gain over the course of a year! We are consuming more calories than we need, so this would be a positive energy balance.

Going forward, consider a diet as a feeding strategy in which you would regulate your calorie intake. One strategy you can use to lose weight is to eat fewer calories. Don't let the fact that fruits and vegetables are healthy fool you into thinking you can munch on them all day. The opposite is true, as you can see. Keep in mind that overall calorie intake is what really counts. Still, these foods contain calories. You can choose the foods you want to eat and calculate how many calories you need based on your weight loss goals using my meal planner.

Many people think they won't be hungry because they drastically reduced the number of calories on their feeding plan. This could happen. However, the hunger pangs can be reduced if you can eat every 2-4 hours.

Divide the number of hours you are awake by three to get a quick formula. If you spend 15 hours a day awake, 5 meals should be your target. Using my meal planner, it was determined that you required 1500 calories total, or an average of 300 calories per meal, for the day. Your chances of success increase thanks to this meal planner.

A meal replacement can help you stay on track if you get busy at work and are unable to eat a meal. Due to the unpredictable nature of life, I do use these frequently throughout the week.

I don't recommend skipping any meals at the beginning of your nutritional plan because doing so might result in what I refer to as "compensating." In essence, because you skipped a meal, you will probably overeat at your next meal psychologically. This will unavoidably result in increased food consumption and weight gain.

Diets generally fail because they are too restrictive for most people. Don't think that all you need to do is consume water and eat vegetables all day. No, that won't work over the long haul.

With my meal planner, you calculate your calorie intake and then create a weekly menu based on the foods you enjoy eating, not what some diet expert says you must consume.

A meal planner helps many people by eliminating the guesswork involved in determining the precise foods they should eat in order to lose weight. What can I eat? is the most frequent query I receive in regards to weight loss. It is now possible to respond to this query.

Rule of thumb

One of the key components to sticking to a diet plan is discipline. It can take months or even years to lose weight through a proper diet and get to your ideal weight. Yo-yo dieting can result from any extreme diet that encourages quick results. Yo-yo dieting is the practice of losing weight while adhering to a diet, only to eventually overeat and gain back the weight lost.

This occurs because the diet he followed was excessively restrictive, banning many food groups and severely restricting his food intake. He can't stick to this diet, so he gives in and eats more. Or it might be the result of a lack of discipline once the desired weight has been reached. This is typically what happens when you follow an extremely high-calorie diet.

In order to prevent that, you should adopt a healthy lifestyle and learn to eat well, exercise frequently, and get enough sleep. It will be challenging at first to break bad habits. But if you follow your new eating strategy for at least 21 to 30 days, it ought to lay a solid groundwork for success.

Your significant other will need to support you as you switch from an unhealthy diet to a healthy one. I've seen it happen far too often where the person who is closest to you will undermine your efforts. Why not convince them to accept your new feeding strategy? Making this change will have a positive impact on their health even if they don't need to lose weight.

The fact that my meal planner has countless possible combinations is the final reason why using one is essential for success. How do I expect you to live on chicken and broccoli every day when I know I couldn't? You won't get bored because of the variety of foods available, including foods you enjoy, and your chances of success will be greatly improved.

Just keep in mind that you can get back on track the following day if you fall off the wagon and consume one or more meals that exceed your daily calorie limit. In the end, all that is required of you is compliance 90% of the time. Obviously, you can't do this every day, but doing it once a week won't significantly hinder your attempts to lose weight.

Trade Secrets

The weight loss industry is keeping a number of things from you and doesn't want you to know them. They are selling fads, devices, and pills to people who are desperate to lose weight, and their business is booming as a result.

Unfortunately, people's wallets are typically the only thing that is getting lighter. Only a small portion of people who buy into one of these methods actually succeed in losing weight and keeping it off. Many of these methods are ineffective.

A few of these business secrets are as follows:

The majority of advertisements for weight loss products deceive the consumer. The vast majority of weight loss products that you hear about on the radio and see on infomercials don't even work as promised. Nevertheless, these products are marketed to consumers with claims such as "Lose the weight and keep it off," "Eat whatever you want," and "no diet or exercise required." In general, if something seems too good to be true, it probably is.

It doesn't necessarily mean something works just because it's "scientifically proven" or "doctor endorsed." These claims are also common, but they never disclose the location or authors of the studies so that you can independently assess their validity.

What does it actually mean, then? These "health professionals" frequently have a financial stake in the product, so they most likely skipped over the scientific research. Even if it was reviewed, they might not have adhered to reasonable review criteria. Why would you want to do something like that and risk your health?

A product's safety for consumers or ability to live up to its promises are not guaranteed simply because the government permits it to be sold. There is a widespread misconception that the government would forbid a product from entering the market if it might endanger you. People frequently believe that the government must first pre-approve them, but this is not always the case.

The safety of products marketed as "natural" or "herbal" cannot be guaranteed. The belief that a product must be safe simply because it contains natural ingredients is another common misconception. However, companies are free to release their products onto the market up until the FDA receives proof that a product is harmful.

You shouldn't believe everything you hear because it may not be true. You should avoid products that make grandiose claims because there are many out there that simply do not live up to their claims.

Likewise, don't believe the claims made by fad diets. Anything that calls for abrupt and drastic changes to your eating habits is very challenging to maintain over time.

They'll start you on a rapid weight-loss cycle, which is always followed by a period during which, in some cases, you'll gain all the weight you lost plus some once your regular eating patterns resume.

Additionally, it makes it even harder the next time you try to lose the weight. These diets have no positive effects on health, and do you really believe that there would be a demand for new ones if they did?

Additionally, you shouldn't rely on the money-back guarantee. The likelihood of getting your money back is about equal to the likelihood that the product will live up to its promises.

Additionally, there isn't a magic cure or quick fix that will enable you to finally lose weight. You can almost certainly guarantee that if a product makes such claims, they won't be true.

CHAPTER TWO:

What Should I Do Now?

You must be dedicated to any diet in order to succeed at it. Only by adopting the proper mindset can you achieve success. Before you can move on to the next phase of your diet, you must first prepare yourself by understanding what stage you are in. It may not be visible, but it is nonetheless present.

Pre-contemplation is the initial stage: You don't think of yourself as overweight. You don't feel like altering who you are. You won't ask for help unless there is a lot of pressure. But if that happened, you wouldn't give in; you'd just give up, feeling defeated by your own situation.

The second is reflection: This is the point at which you admit that you have a weight problem and begin to consider a solution. However, you are unwilling to implement that remedy. Knowing what steps to take to effect a change, but never being ready to do so, you would simply think about it. You will put off implementing the solution.

The third is planning: You've finally made up your mind to address your weight issue. You stop dwelling on your issue and start identifying the solution. Additionally, you would begin to envision a time in the future when you are thinner and feel much better. However, you aren't yet fully committed at this point. Even so, you might still be on the fence about the solution because it calls for a lifestyle adjustment.

Action is the fourth: You begin to take steps toward losing weight. You would begin making food choices and engaging in daily exercise. It is the first step toward achieving your specific objective. Setting goals is a must when trying to lose weight. It's very likely that your entire diet plan won't go as you had hoped if you don't set your goals.

Describe the following:

- **What is your current situation right now?** In order to lose weight, make a list of all your eating habits, food preferences, and other factors. exercising, etc.
- **What motivates your desire to lose weight?** This might be for a forthcoming occasion, the summer, or even for a special someone. Write down the one, biggest reason that comes to mind.
- **What advantages do you gain from losing weight?** As many as you can list. Health, more

energy, a partner's admiration, etc. are some examples. This should be your primary driving force.

- **Your Objective**. Write this in bold to help it really stick in your mind: "I want to lose XX pounds of weight in XX days." Personally, I think it's unrealistic to set a goal of more than 10 pounds every two weeks, especially if you're trying to achieve it for the first time. Be sensible. You must use the verb "want" instead of "wish."

Record everything on paper, then review it frequently. Placing it where you can see it will help. You will be constantly reminded of WHY you do this and what the benefits are once you start seeing it every day.

Once you start, don't give up because it won't be simple.

Stepping Out of Your Comfort Zone

Consider your motivation for not actually wanting to lose weight if you find yourself coming up with justifications rather than STARTING an efficient diet. You must possess the ability to push past your comfort zone and, in the words of Nike's catchphrase, "JUST DO IT!"

Maintenance would be the last step. You must maintain the momentum you had during the action stage. If at any point you stop being dedicated or supportive, you will revert to any of the earlier stages.

The final stage of your diet plan is therefore the most crucial because you need to maintain your commitment over an extended period of time. There are several strategies you can employ to maintain your commitment.

Make a list of your initial motivations for doing this before anything else. To keep your focus on your goals, review the list every day. Avoid thinking anything unfavorable. Never use words like "never" or "depriving" in your vocabulary. You are only having desserts "occasionally and in moderation" rather than "never." As a result, the word "deprived" can be changed to "choosing" since you have decided to forego chocolate cakes.

Imagine in your mind's eye a slimmer version of yourself accomplishing all the things you have always desired. Your determination to stick with this plan and be determined to succeed will be boosted by this visualization. Every day, each time you wake up and whenever you feel your commitment waning, perform this visualization.

Who to Approach When You Want to Lose Weight?

You should involve some other people in your weight loss journey now that you've made the decision to lose weight. These people can assist you in a variety of ways, including selecting a diet strategy, establishing goals, and providing you with motivation as you move forward.

A dietician: A dietician will have a broad base of knowledge that can assist you in understanding your body and preparing a diet that will meet your individual needs because, in the majority of states and countries, obtaining a medical license is a prerequisite for becoming a dietician. Meal planners are a less expensive option to dieticians. My meal planner is a revolutionary new system that has a patent pending. It assists you in building completely balanced diets using your favorite foods by working with you as if they were your own personal dietician or nutritionist.

An individual trainer: Most people have never been taught how to exercise properly. This, in my opinion, is very crucial if you've never engaged in any sort of weight training. I wouldn't sign a long-term contract with a trainer, and I'd want them to know my objectives and how they plan to support me in achieving them. I would caution you that for at least the first year, you must scale the workouts in terms of weight and duration.

Family and friends: I always dislike doing this, but I have a plan that I believe you can put to use quickly.

I detested telling people whenever I embarked on one of my 100 diets. Because this was yet another diet I was starting, I thought they were judging me. Instead, say (if they ask) that you're just trying to eat a little healthier and that you're done with diets when you're at the dinner table during a party, holiday, or other special occasion.

Persisting Through Failure

You will inevitably fail when attempting to lose weight or keep it off because you are only human. People who are successful at losing weight did not give up when things got difficult; instead, they persevered and discovered a lesson.

The two main strategies for handling failure are to Keep trying and picking things up.

Don't worry about the little things if you stray from your diet or skip an exercise day. Don't allow it to stop you. Get it out of your head. Consider all of your good days rather than just one mistake. The more healthy lifestyle choices you make, the more good days you have; before you know it, the bad days are few and far between. But the key is to persevere and get through the difficult times. Consider it a cheat day, then move on. This is how you persevere; it's okay to fail for a day, just don't let it turn into a week, then a month.

To deal with failures, you must learn to accept them as a natural part of life.

The next step is to take lessons from your errors. It is frequently more effective to learn from your mistakes than from your successes.

When you fail, view it as a teaching moment. Just like in business, when you try something and fail, you learn what doesn't work.

The same holds true for losing weight. Perhaps you should abstain from drinking if you find that every time you drink, your new diet suffers. Reschedule your workout if you find that you consistently skip it on Fridays due to a late work meeting.

Along with death and taxes, failure is a given in life. Even if you could, you wouldn't want to because you can't avoid it. Your failures and successes both teach you valuable lessons about life. Don't be afraid of failing; just keep trying and keep learning.

Buddy System

Adding some accountability to your routine is one of the best things you can do when trying to lose weight. How do you go about that?

The Buddy System

A great motivator is having a friend with whom to attempt weight loss. When you actually tell someone about your weight loss goals, you will feel more responsible for achieving them. They can also be useful because the person can understand your difficulties with weight loss. You can encourage one another by sharing both your victories and your setbacks.

A workout partner is invaluable if you exercise frequently. They can transform a dull jog or walk into a therapy session that also serves as exercise. Bringing a friend along for a hike in the wilderness is always more enjoyable!

Having a friend is also beneficial if you enjoy weightlifting. You guys can push each other while also encouraging and helping each other out with things like spots on heavy lifts.

The sad truth is that you can probably find a weight loss buddy in your circle of friends today. Don't worry if you can't; you can always do it virtually online.

The bottom line is that working with a friend can help with accountability, support, and motivation if you're trying to lose weight. Now go find your weight-loss partner!

Why It's Important to keep a Daily Schedule

Setting up a daily training schedule is the following step in planning your weight loss objectives. Personally, I find that 6AM is a good time for me.

It was challenging to wake up so early at first, but eventually it became a habit. I'll list a few benefits of exercising at this time of day.

1) You have completed your daily exercise.

2) You have the afternoon free to spend with your family, partner, friends, etc.

3) It's okay if you are delayed at work because your workout is already finished.

But those are the reasons I train at this hour of the morning. Friends of mine have admitted to favoring the late afternoon and early evening. Once more, the time doesn't really matter as much as the fact that you must complete the task.

Maintaining Your Balance: You're more likely to stick to your goals when you have a set schedule to follow, so record everything in a journal or other journaling tool like a smartphone. However, if you do skip a workout or have an extra snack, you can note it and resolve to do better the following time.

Understanding Your Daily Routine: It can help to have a written schedule of when you should exercise or eat your meals so that you are prepared. In this way you can schedule things around your workout times, rather than scheduling over them and just missing workouts altogether.

This is simple to do, and once you start doing it, you'll find that you miss your workouts more frequently until you completely lose track of your fitness goals.

Lose More Weight: By sticking to a schedule, you are more likely to complete your workouts on time and ultimately lose more weight (or very, very few in the long run).

You will find it much more difficult to maintain a consistent rate of weight loss if you frequently switch between diets, skip workouts, or skip meals, which confuses your body's metabolism.

CHAPTER THREE

Healthy Nutrition and Its Benefits

You may have heard a lot of people say that eating a healthy diet is essential for maintaining a healthy body, but you need to understand what healthy nutrition actually entails and why it is so crucial. Define nutrition first.

"Nutrition is the process of giving your body all the essential nutrients that will enable it to develop in a healthy and balanced manner."

This is the simplest definition of nutrition, and it informs you that you must consume healthy foods that are rich in essential nutrients. Your body can become strong and healthy with proper nutrition, and it can also grow and heal on its own. While a poor nutrition plan can weaken your body, make you ill, and prevent you from fighting off some minor illnesses.

Calories In - Calories Out

Most people who want to lose weight have experimented with a variety of diets, supplements, and/or plans. There are many different weight loss strategies that can be purchased. They're all making outrageous claims.

The harsh reality is that there are no magic pills, diets, or exercise equipment that will make weight vanish overnight. It all comes down to eating properly, maintaining good health, and consuming fewer calories than you expend.

That is the origin of the proverb "calories in, calories out." Make sure you expend more calories (out) than you take in (in).

This is a naive way of thinking, and a healthy diet involves more than just counting calories. We'll examine that in later chapters, but for now, let's focus on establishing a calorie deficit.

You'll need some basic information to track this. You must first determine how many calories you naturally burn each day. It all comes down to things like weight and age.

How to Determine How Many Calories You Burn Each Day

Men's BMR calculation (kg) BMR is calculated as follows: 66.5 + 13.75 x weight in kg + 5.003 x height in cm - (6.755 x age in years)

Men's BMR calculation (pounds) BMR is calculated as follows: 66 + 6.23 x weight in pounds + 12.7 x height in inches - (6.76 x age in years)

Female BMR calculation (kg) BMR is calculated as follows: 655.1 + (9.563 x weight in kg) + 1.850 x height in cm - (4.676 x age in years)

BMR for women is calculated as follows: BMR = 655 + 4.35 times weight in pounds + 4.7 times height in inches - (4.7 x age in years)

This equation will show you how many calories you burn each day just from breathing, heartbeat, etc. These are the calories you would burn if you remained stationary all day (basal metabolic rate).

Once you know that figure, you must begin keeping track of the calories you consume and burn. There is a lot of information to keep track of, which makes this challenging. It's not about starving yourself or working out nonstop until you pass out. It all comes down to being conscious of what you put into and exert from your body. Even though losing weight can be challenging, if you can control your intake and expenditure of calories, you can succeed!

Clean Eating

The fundamental weight loss principle, calories in versus calories out, has already been discussed. It is a fundamental tip because you still need to be cautious about where you are getting your calories from. It's probably not a good idea to consume two corndogs per day in order to reduce your calorie intake.

Although there is no official definition for the phrase "eating clean," it generally refers to eating whole, wholesome foods and avoiding processed foods and refined sugars.

While it may not always be possible to consume only "clean" foods, if you are getting the majority of your calories from these foods, you are doing great.

Fast food and junk food are automatically eliminated from your diet when you eat clean because you avoid processed foods. Don't worry if you consume some processed food; the goal is to consume as little of it as possible.

Here are some general guidelines for eating healthy:

Read labels carefully: Read the ingredients and nutritional information on every product you purchase.

whenever possible, choose whole grains: Whole grain doesn't always equate to whole wheat, either!

Frequently consume fruits and vegetables: They are excellent sources of healthy whole calories.

Don't buy microwaveable meals, eat out less, and prepare more of your own meals. Even though they are marketed as "healthy," these meals can be very high in sodium.

When cooking, choose lean meats: It's okay to eat meat because the protein will help you feel satisfied and build muscle. Excellent meat options include fish and chicken.

Steer clear of processed meats like hot dogs and bologna.

Whole nuts that are unsalted or lightly salted can take the place of junk food.

Visit these free websites for fantastic clean recipes: http://easy-stir-fry-recipes.com and http://low-carb-chickenrecipes.com

Don't worry about slacking off; allow yourself the occasional cheat day.

It can be challenging to eat healthily while out, but more eateries are starting to offer this option. If you're really hungry, you might need to add some protein to a salad, though!

A great way to ensure that you are healthy overall and that you lose weight is to eat cleanly. You don't have to try to turn on a switch and make the transition overnight, but it isn't always simple. Clean up your diet if you're serious about losing weight and improving your health.

Water Is Your Best Friend

According to research, you should drink at least 8 glasses of water each day, but how much you actually need will depend on your weight. Your weight would need to be divided by 2. Therefore, a man weighing 180 pounds would require 90 ounces of water per day.

So why is water recommended by experts and why is it thought to be so vital to living a healthy life?

First off, it aids in the removal of waste products, which prevents dehydration and maintains the kidneys' good health. Additionally, it helps to speed up metabolism, which aids in weight loss.

But in addition to paying attention to what experts advise, you should prioritize paying attention to your body. Naturally, you will drink water to rehydrate yourself when you are thirsty.

Depending on the type of work you do, you should try to develop the habit of regularly drinking water or, even better, keeping a water bottle on hand. This is especially important on extremely hot days because the heat causes you to perspire and your body loses water, so you will need to rehydrate.

Water has a crucial role in our lives because of this. In addition to having no calories, it is also the best and healthiest way to quench your thirst. In the long run, you might think about replacing fruit drinks and sodas with water at every meal to help reduce your calorie intake. You'll also feel much better without the extra sugar that comes with the other drinks.

CHAPTER FOUR

The Importance of Exercise

In this chapter I'm going to tell you what works best for melting fat like butter on a hot stove.

Exercising

First of all, the human body is built for movement. Exercise has many advantages besides the obvious ones of keeping a healthy body weight.

1) Fights illness;

2) Elevates your mood;

3) Increases your energy;

4) Aids in better sleep; and

5) Better sex as well

Seven out of ten adults, or nearly four out of ten, are not physically active on a regular basis, according to a recent survey. You run the risk of developing heart disease, diabetes, and stroke if you don't exercise. About 300,000 people have died as a result of this.

You should speak with a doctor before beginning an exercise program. If you've been sitting on the couch and not working out for a while, this is crucial.

There are many different perspectives on fat loss in the world today. Running is typically the first exercise activity people do. In any case, it increases your heart rate and is also aerobic.

What burns the most fat is aerobic exercise, right? You might be surprised to learn that running isn't actually that effective at burning fat. That's because once your body has become conditioned by the exercise, you frequently reach a plateau (Peele, 2010).

In contrast, I've discovered a technique that guarantees you never plateau by steadily increasing the demands with each workout. Additionally, it burns fat up to 3,000% more effectively than your morning run!

Why HIIT is Better Than Running

It is an original strategy and is known as HIIT, or High Intensity Interval Training. It will cut the length of your workouts and burn up to nine times more fat than running (Cossaboon). That means it is 36 times more effective overall when combined with the fact that it completes in a quarter the time. How is this even conceivable?

First off, you burn more calories because of the intensity of the workout itself. You come out ahead even though a smaller portion of these come exclusively from fat because the total is higher.

The most astounding aspect of HIIT training is, however, the second way it functions. Your metabolism is increased for up to 24 hours after your workout is over. That implies that while you're lounging on your couch at 11 p.m. the same night, you could be burning fat!

HIIT was a great fit for me because I value getting the most out of my money. Additionally, you only need to exercise three times per week to start seeing results; you don't even need to exercise every day.

How Does it Work?

The HIIT technique employs a two-pronged strategy to produce results quickly. You will use two different intensities during your workout rather than maintaining one intensity the entire time.

Running at a respectable pace is a good example of the first, which is a moderate level. The second is short bursts of high intensity, like sprinting at your top speed.

You should train at a slower pace for two to five minutes, followed by a quick burst of high intensity exercise lasting 10 to thirty seconds. Repeat this template once more while returning to the moderate level when 15 to 20 minutes have passed.

Your metabolism will be in overdrive at the conclusion, and it may remain that way for several hours or even the rest of the day. This means that while you exercise and while your body is recovering afterward, you are both burning fat. This will accelerate your results and start melting the fat off of your frame immediately.

Stay In the Zone

But if you don't keep your heart rate up high enough during your fat loss routine, you won't experience any of these wonderful advantages.

What rate should you aim for to get the most out of HIIT? Your heart rate should be close to your safe limit during the brief times when you are working as hard as you can.

How can you come to this conclusion? First, subtract your age from 220 to determine your maximum heart rate. Then, when you are in the high intensity part of your HIIT session, you should aim for 85% of this number (Baker, 2011).

To hit the beats per minute required to produce the desired effect, you'll need to work harder than you probably imagine. You haven't worked yourself hard enough if you can still talk while doing this or if you aren't gasping for air afterward.

Melt the Fat Away

You'll have a potent tool to aid you in your weight loss program when you use HIIT in conjunction with your target heart rate. Incorporating this kind of exercise into your fat loss routine will hasten your progress and improve your outcomes!

Since HIIT enables you to go even further than traditional cardio training, it is a more effective method for burning fat. You see, the brief periods of intense exercise are designed to push you close to your limit each time.

Since you can't sustain this level for the duration of a workout, your energy expenditure will inevitably drop.

For instance, you might be able to sprint at your top speed for ten to fifteen seconds, but not for the entire thirty minute workout. You have to slow down to a fast run to get through the workout, which has different effects on your body.

Add Kettlebell Strength Training to Your Routine

Strength training with kettlebells is a useful supplement to your HIIT workouts. Women avoid the weight room, while many men rush to the gym. You may believe that doing this kind of exercise will make you look bulky and muscle-bound rather than give you the lean appearance you desire.

However, weight lifting with kettlebells is very effective for weight loss when done properly. You will maintain your flexibility while also developing lean muscle with the exercise I've included, giving you a nice athletic look.

In addition to being advantageous for other reasons, load-bearing exercise has been shown to prevent osteoporosis (Rogers, 2012). For your lower body, you can achieve this benefit by simply walking, but for your upper body, you must lift weights to achieve the same bone-building effects.

Additionally, resistance training can increase your metabolism for several hours following your workout, which will further your weight loss efforts. Women must utilize the weight room and the potent kettlebell to the fullest in order to achieve all of these benefits.

Why Use a Kettlebell for Exercise? A good question. I didn't fully understand it the first time I saw someone train with one. But after being asked to take part in a workout, I was able to appreciate just how useful these little tips could be for getting in shape.

Unless you've been living in a cave in Afghanistan, you've probably heard that kettlebells are Russian in origin and that the fitness industry has welcomed them with open arms.

Let's talk about the many benefits of training with kettlebells:

- Strengthening and muscular endurance
- No gym membership is necessary;
- you can work out inside or outside;
- you can burn fat and lose weight;
- you can build lean muscle;
- you can develop mental toughness;
- you can develop a strong core and sexy abs.

Choosing the Right Kettlebell

When beginning any kettlebell exercise program, this is a crucial choice. Women should start with an 18-pound kettlebell and men with a 35-pound bell. In the beginning these weights should get you off on the right foot and when the workouts are done with the proper intensity they are plenty heavy.

Security First

I've said it before, but it's crucial that you speak with your doctor before beginning any physical fitness regimen. Despite the kettlebell's relative "lightness," using it incorrectly can still result in injury. It's also crucial to warm up properly before beginning any of the exercises in this book. Start out slowly and get familiar with the fundamentals.

Footwear

When using a kettlebell, it's crucial to keep your feet flat on the ground at all times. Wearing "running" shoes with a raised heel is not advised. You might get hurt if you don't stand correctly as a result of this. To save a few dollars, you can wear minimalist footwear or simply go barefoot.

Getting better with practice

I appreciate your desire to get started training and your determination to work toward getting the body you deserve. But for the first week, the only thing I want you to do is watch the videos that go along with it; after that, I really want you to practice the kettlebell swing.

The swing is the most crucial move that I still work on, and while I don't aim for perfection, I do try to maintain proper form.

You can find my suggested kettlebell workout in the following chapter. This is complete with pictures and directions for carrying out each day's exercise.

Kettlebell Workout Routine

No matter if you've ever used a kettlebell or not, be sure to pick a weight that you can move without getting hurt. Kettlebells are an excellent tool for getting in shape, but they must be handled with care. You will see results from this workout after eight weeks if you follow a healthy diet and get enough rest. Prior to beginning any exercise program, be sure to get your doctor's approval.

The exercise is intended to be performed four days per week. Mon./Tues., Wednesday as a rest day, and then Thursday/Friday are my suggestions. Life happens, of course. As closely as you can, follow the plan.

Each workout's outline is provided below, followed by more thorough instructions.

Front Plank

The starting position is on your hands and knees with the back flat. Contract the abdominal muscles. Without rotating the trunk or sagging or arching the spine, elevate yourself into the push up position with your weight on your forearms and toes. Keep your head up looking forward. The goal is to hold this position for 60 seconds. If you cannot hold for 1 minute, then repeat until 1 minute has elapsed. Continue to breathe when conducting this exercise.

The Hip Flexor Stretch

Movement:

1. Start with left knee on the ground, and right leg up with both arms over head.

2. Hold for approximately 10 seconds.

3. Switch to the other side and hold for 10 seconds.

Note: This warm-up exercise promotes stretching out the core, hip flexors, back, quadriceps, lats, and is just an overall great stretch to loosen up. This is perhaps the best overall stretch you can do before any physical event.

Push-Up

I realize most people think they know how to perform a push-up.

Movement:

1. Bend the elbows, lowering your body until your upper arms are parallel with the ground.

2. Fully extend your arms so that your elbows are "locked" out.

The key is to fully extend in the up position with your arms locked out. Secondly, make sure that when you are in the down position your arms are parallel to the ground. Don't think fast here, do them slow and controlled for full effect of this movement.

Variation: If you are unable to perform a push-up as illustrated, assume a stance on your knees to perform them correctly. This is a natural progression.

Kettlebell Swing

Movement:

1. Squat down with your back straight and lift up the weight. Don't confuse this with a vertical back, simply keep it straight. Don't round your back.

2. Squat up and stand erect with your shoulders back.

3. Think sit back rather than dip down.

4. Ensure that your hips are extended as well as your knees at the top with your body in a straight line.

5. For the Russian style swing illustrated here the bell should never go above parallel.

6. Ensure that you are either barefoot or wearing a minimalist shoe so that you are flat footed.

Precautions: Work with light weight initially until you can perform the movement correctly.

Turkish Get-Up

Movement:

1. Use both of your hands while in a fetal position to lift the kettlebell from the ground at the start of the movement and at the completion of the movement.

2. Next you want to set the foot and hand. Notice that the arm on the kettlebell side is vertical with a straight wrist. The knee on the side of the kettlebell is bent to prepare you for eventually standing up. Both the lats and your core are engaged and ready for work. The arm opposite the kettlebell is positioned 45 degrees and your opposite leg is straight.

3. Lock your elbow and keep it locked for the duration of the movement.

4. Keep your shoulder in a "packed" position at all times during the movement.

5. Get up smoothly and slowly and concentrate on each position.

6. This is not an exercise performed rapidly.

Precaution: This looks deceivingly easy. Use a very light weight (5lbs) or even a sneaker until you hit each position. In my Hardstyle Kettlebell Certification course, we used the sneaker. I highly suggest the sneaker.

Deadlift

Movement:

1. Straddle the bell with your feet a little wider than shoulder-width.

2. Squat down with arms extended downward between your legs and grab the bell's handle with both hands.

3. Ensure that your shoulders are over the bell and keep your back straight.

4. Pull the bell off the floor by extending your hips and knees ensuring your chest is up.

5. Lower the bell while squatting down and keeping your back taunt with a vertical back.

Precaution: Ensure you do not round your back. Ensure you can do an air squat with no weight properly before adding any weight.

Snatch

Movement:

1. Begin with the Russian Style swing.

2. Catch the bell softly without "banging" the bell on your wrist.

3. You can do this by "punching" to the top of the movement.

4. When you lock out at the top, your arm should be level with your head.

5. Lower the bell down to complete a swing and repeat as needed.

Precaution: Keep back straight, work with a weight you can safely control.

Learning the Rack

Movement:

1. Pick up the bell with 1 hand

2. Use your 2nd hand to get the bell into position

3. Now you are in the rack position or where the clean ends up

4. Drop the bell down by moving your hips backwards and "sitting down"

5. The bell is moving completely vertically down by moving your hips back and not pushing the bell forward.

Precaution: Keep your back straight, use a weight that is lighter until you learn the movement.

The Rack

Movement:

1. Stand over the kettlebells. Take a deep breath and hold and pull back between legs.
2. As the kettlebells come back (breathe in), bend slightly at the knees, pushing your hips backwards

allowing the kettlebells to pass between your legs. Ensure back is straight.

3. Using your glutes like a rubber band, open your hips and propel the bell forward. As you drive through with your hips (breathe out) until you come to a triple extension. The bells should land between your arms and forearms, with elbow tucked throughout move.

4. Your bells are now in a racked position.

Precaution: Ensure your back is straight, and select a weight that is within your ability to safely lift the weight.

Double Kettlebell Front Squat

Movement:

1. Begin with the bells in the racked position.

2. Set handles just above your collar bone.

3. Have your feet a little wider than shoulder-width apart.

4. Inhale as you sit down while keeping your back straight.

5. Exhale on the way up and stand tall.

Precautions: Do not round your back. Ensure your back is straight. Select a weight you can safely move.

Clean

Movement:

1. Straddle the bell with your feet a little more than shoulder width apart.

2. Your elbow should be part of your torso.

3. Your hips will do all of the work.

4. Make the bell travel in a straight line; which is the shortest distance between 2 objects.

5. Do not dip your knees when receiving or "racking" the bell.

6. Avoid banging your wrist or forearm.

Precautions: Back straight, choose a weight that you can work with safely.

Press

Movement:

1. Stand with your feet slightly wider than shoulder width.

2. Take the bell from the rack or clean it from the floor and position in front of chest with the bell against the outside of your arm.

3. Press the bell up until your arm is fully extended overhead.

4. Lower to the front of your chest.

Precaution: Ensure that you are utilizing a weight that will enable you perform the move properly.

Overhead or Waiters Walk

Movement:

1. Begin with the bell in the press out position.

2. Ensure that your shoulder and elbow are in a "locked" position.

3. Begin walking.

Precautions: Make sure you have a clear path (obviously), select your weight carefully

Suitcase Carry

Movement:

1. Pick up the bell as you would a suitcase deadlift before carrying.

2. Keep the shoulders level and core tight with no compensation from one side to another.

3. A heavier weight may be required to reach the desired effect.

Precautions: Ensure you your back is straight and not rounded when picking up or setting down the weight. As always, select a weight you can move safely.

Rack Walk

Movement:

1. Begin with the bells in the racked position.

2. Ensure that the handles are above your collar bones.

3. Keep the bells next to your bicep.

4. Do not let the bells droop or sag.

5. Start walking.

Precautions: Ensure your walking path is free of obstacles and select a weight you can safely move with.

Goblet Squat

Movement:

1. Grab the bell by the horns.

2. Feet shoulder width apart or a little more than shoulder width apart.

3. Pull yourself down.

4. Keep your chest up while keeping your back as straight as possible.

5. Elbows come inside your knees with the weight on your heels and not toes.

6. Stand straight up.

Precautions: Do no round the back and select a weight appropriate for your abilities.

Single Arm Deadlift

Movement:

1. Performed like deadlift but with weight to your side.

2. Bell will be even with your ankle.

3. Bend at the waist and knees while your back is straight.

4. Stand straight up without compensating for the side with no weight.

5. Stand straight up.

Precautions: Back must be straight and not rounded. Select a weight for your abilities in order to lift safely.

Farmers Walk

Movement:

Performed like a standard deadlift but with 2 bells at your side. Use heavier weights so the movement is challenging. Begin walking for the prescribed time.

Precautions: Do not round your back and always select a weight you can safely move.

Hand to Hand Swing

Movement:

1. Begin with regular swing except now you will release the bell at the top of the swing.

2. Grab the bell with your other hand.

3. Move with a purpose.

Precautions: If the bell is too far forward when you go to grab it let it go and reset. Choose a weight that you can safely move.

Hand to Hand Snatch

Movement:

1. Begin the movement by doing the snatch with a swing.

2. Move the bell back down with the same hand.

3. Swing the bell back up and receive the bell with the other hand.

4. Move the bell back down and begin the transition as required.

Precautions: Ensure you do not round your back and select a weight that you can safely move.

Month 1

Day 1

TGU- 3 each side alternating

Overhead kb walk: 30 seconds each side

KB deadlift 4x5 choose weight, focus on hinge and lockout

Swing ladders- 3 bells of different sizes, 8 reps each x4

Suitcase carry- 3 sets of: 30 heavier bell

Single arm deadlift 4x5 each arm

Single arm swings- 4x8 each side

Plank 5x: 30

Detailed Explanation:

TGU-3 ea. Side alternating. Here you want to focus on hitting each position in the move. Do the left side then right side until you do a total of 6 TGU. Work with a weight you can safely handle. This is not a move that is done fast, but rather an intentional movement. There is nothing wrong with using even something as light as your sneaker for the first 2 weeks, to learn the movement.

O/H KB Walk 30 seconds each side. Choose your weight carefully here. You are going to move with the weight overhead for a total of 30 seconds. Ensure that you lock that arm which is overhead. Walk normally.

Kettlebell Dead Lift 4 x 5. Choose an appropriate weight, focus on the hinge and lockout. When it is written 4 x 5 you will do 4 sets of 5. There is no pre-determined rest period here. If you choose a weight that isn't too light or too heavy, you'll most likely only need to rest 1 minute.

Swing Ladders-3 bells of different sizes, 8 Reps x 4. If you are just beginning to use kettlebells, start light. For men a 35# bell is probably the max and women a 25# bell. Start with the lightest weight do 8 two handed swings, then move to the middle weight and do 8 two handed swings, and then move to the heaviest weight and do 8 two handed swings. You will then rest and do it again 3 more times.

Suitcase Carry: 3 sets of 30 seconds. I would use my non-dominate hand first, then dominant, then non-dominate. If you need to rest, simply set the weight down, rest and resume.

Single Arm Deadlift 4 x 5 each arm. Focus on not compensating with the arm that is not picking the weight up. Ensure your back is straight. Do 5 reps on one arm, then 5 reps with the other arm. Rest required amount, and repeat 3 additional times. Choose a challenging weight here.

Single Arm Swings 4 x 8 each side. Start with either arm, 8 with one arm, 8 with the other arm, rest as needed and do 3 more times. Ensure you select a weight you can safely move.

Plank 5 x :30 seconds. Chances are you won't be able to hold the plank for 30 seconds. That's ok, if you can only do 10 seconds, rest do 10

Day 2

TGU- pause in each position for 5 seconds, 2 each side

2 hand swings 5x10

Hip flexor stretch

1 hand swing 8L and 8 R 6 goblet squats

Repeat 1 hand swings and goblets x4

Hand to hand swings

Do 20 swings, go into: 30 plank repeat x4

Farmers walk 4 sets of: 30 to: 45 seconds

Detailed Explanation:

Turkish Get-Up Pause in ea. Position 5 seconds, 2 ea. Side. Here you will pause on your forearm, palm, knee, and in standing, and do the same on the way down. Focus on really feeling each position. Ensure you are selecting a light weight. There is nothing wrong with using even something as light as your sneaker for the first 2 weeks, to learn the movement.

2 Hand Swings 5 x 10. You will do 10 repetitions with a weight you can safely handle. Rest for a short time, then do this 4 more times.

Hip Flexor Stretch. Really take time to stretch each side. Focus on the entire body here.

1 Hand Swing 8L & 8R/6 Goblet Squats. You will do 8 swings with your left hand, then 8 with your right hand, and with same weight move right into doing 6 goblet squats. Rest for less than a minute and repeat 3 more times.

Do 20 hand to hand swings, then 30 seconds in the plank. Ensure that you've practiced this movement before doing it for the first time. If you are doing this in your house, make sure there is nothing that can be broken is in the way. If the bell gets away from you, let it go, and start over. Once you do 20 hand to hand swings, you will immediately do 30 seconds in the plank and immediately commence with the 20 hand to hand swings. You will do this for a total of 4 rounds.

Farmers Walk-4 sets of 30 seconds to 45 seconds. Choose a heavy enough weight so it is challenging, but not so heavy you have to set it down after 15 seconds. Once you hit between 30 and 45 seconds, set the weight down, recover, and repeat 3 more times.

Day 3

TGU to the standing position, walk for: 30 seconds then come down, repeat on way down

KB deadlift- 4x5

KB swings 30/30 for 10 minutes

Goblet squat 6 reps, at the bottom of the 6th rep curl the kb 6 times by the horns, repeat 4 times

30/30 1 arm swings. Swing L then rest for: 30, repeat for 8 minutes

Hip flexor stretch

Detailed Explanation:

Turkish Get-Up Standing Position Walk 30 seconds then come down, repeat for other arm. Do a Turkish get-up, then walk for 30 seconds, stop, come down, switch arms, and repeat.

Kettlebell Deadlift 4 x 5. Do 5 Repetitions with a weight that isn't light, but not too heavy that you cannot complete 4 sets. Once you do 5 reps, rest for approximately 1 minute, and then do 3 more times. Ensure that your back is straight, and breathe in on the way down, and out on the way up.

Kettlebell Swings 30/30 for 10 minutes. You will do 30 seconds of 2 arm swings, rest for 30 seconds and do this for a total of 10 minutes.

Goblet Squat 6 Reps, @ bottom of the 6th Rep, curl the kettlebell 6x by the horns. Repeat 4x. So you will do 6 goblet squats, sit in the squat, then do 6 bicep curls with the bell. Do this for 3 more times. Don't be too aggressive with the weight here. Select a weight that you can curl vs. a weight that you can do a goblet squat with.

Hip Flexor Stretch. Really focus on a solid total body stretch here. Try to accumulate 20 seconds on each side. I love this stretch!

Day 4

TGU, alternate each side for a total of 10 minutes

10 2 handed swings

8R and 8L 1 arm swings

10 goblet squats

20 hand to hand swings

:30 overhead walk L/R

:30 suitcase carry L/R

Repeat 4-6 times above for time

Detailed Explanation:

Turkish Get-Up, Alt ea. Side for a total of 10 minutes. Be careful with weight selection here as you will continuously be moving arm to arm and doing the get up.

Do not focus on speed. Feel each step in order to perform this movement correctly.

10 two handed Swings

8R & 8L 1 Arm Swings

10 Goblet Squats

20 Hand to Hand Swings

30 second overhead walk L/R

30 second suitcase carry L/R

Repeat 4-6 times for time

The goal on this day is to move from exercise to exercise without resting. Once you complete on round, then rest, recharge, and set a goal to complete 4 to 6 rounds.

Month 2

Day 1

TGU- use a heavier bell if possible 6 total, 3 per side alternating

1 swing, 1 snatch into overhead walk for :15

2 swing, 2 snatch into overhead walk for :15

3 swing, 3 snatch into overhead walk for

:15 4 swing, 4 snatch into overhead walk for

:15 Repeat above x5

Goblet squat- pause at bottom position for :5 then come up. 5x5

Kb rack walk

5 sets of :30

Detailed Explanation:

Turkish Get-Up Use a heavier bell if possible. Doing a total of 6, 3 each side alternating. Now that you've been doing the program for a month, you should be able to do more weight. Obviously, select a weight that is safe for your ability.

1 Swing, 1 Snatch into Overhead Walk for 15 Seconds

2 Swings, 2 Snatches into Overhead Walk for 15 Seconds

3 Swings, 3 Snatches into Overhead Walk for 15 Seconds

4 Swings, 4 Snatches into Overhead Walk for 15 Seconds

Repeat above for a total of 5 times

Here is how the workout works: You will do a swing, a snatch, walk for 15 seconds, then do this through 4 swings/snatches then rest as needed, and do 4 more times. Keep the rest period as short as possible. Really push yourself here.

Goblet Squat-Pause at Bottom position for 5 seconds then come up 5 x 5. Here you will do 1 goblet squat, sit at the bottom position for 5 seconds, come up and do this for 5 times. Rest as needed, and then do 4 more times.

Kettlebell Rack Walks 5 sets of 30 seconds: Rack the weight, and simply walk for 30 seconds. Keep rest short, then do 4 more times.

Day 2

TGU 8 minutes total, alternate each side

Clean and press 5x5

Double kb front squat 5x5

Push-up 4 sets of perfect form 20 swings,

20 hand to hand swings,

:30 rack walk.

repeat x4

Detailed Explanation:

Turkish Get-Up 8 minutes total, Alternating each side. Just a reminder here, don't focus on speed, focus on movement throughout the Get-up. A slightly heavier weight that you can safely handle will cause your core to get some extra work!

Clean & Press 5 x 5. Do a Clean, then press it and do this for 5 repetitions, rest, then do 4 more times. You will be able to clean much more than you can press. Base the weight off of your press here on this movement.

Double Kettlebell Front Squat 5 x 5. Ensure you rack the weight, keep your back straight, do 5 reps rest and do 4 more times. Choose your weight wisely.

Push-Ups 4 sets of perfect form. This is truly a test of your mental strength. Do as many push-ups as you can with perfect form, rest, and do 3 more times. Record the number of push-ups, so the next 3 weeks you will know if you are progressing. Focus on form here NOT speed. Really push yourself here.

20 Swings, 20 Hand to Hand Swings, 30 seconds Rack Walk, repeat 4x. You should try to use the same weight for this. So do 20 two handed swings, then 20 hand to hand swings, and lastly rack walk for 30 seconds, rest as needed and do 3 more times. Try to keep the rest period short.

Day 3

Overhead walk 4x :30 each arm

suitcase carry 4x:30 each arm

10 1 arm swings L/R

10 snatches L/R 20 hand to hand snatches

repeat x4

2 hand swings, 8 minutes total 40/20

Detailed Explanation:

Overhead Walk 4 x 30 seconds each arm

Suitcase Carry 4 x 30 seconds each arm

10 1 Arm Swings Left then Right

10 Snatches Left then Right

20 Hand to Hand Snatches

Repeat 4x

Move from exercise to exercise without resting. You should know how to do hand to hand snatches before attempting here. After a round is completed, rest for a short period, catch your breath, and do 3 more times. Really push yourself here!

Then:

2 Hand Swings @ 40/20, 8 minutes total. A real test here, do 40 seconds of 2 handed swings, rest 20 seconds and do a total of 8 times.

Day 4

TGU each arm

20 2 handed swings

10 R and 10L 1 arm swings

8 goblet squats

8L and 8R snatches

2 TGU each arm

Rack walks :30 Repeat 4-6 times for time.

Detailed Explanation:

1 Turkish Get-Up each Arm. Challenge yourself here!

20 2 Handed Swings

10 Right and 10 Left 1 Arm swings

8 Goblet Squats

8 Left & 8 Right Snatches

2 Turkish Get-Ups Each Arm

Rack Walks 30 seconds

 Repeat 4-6 times for time.

Notes: The Get-ups are not to be done fast. Feel each position. Move from exercise to exercise with a weight that is challenging, rest and aim for 4 to 6 sets.

If you've completed 8 weeks of the training program, you can always, start back at week 1 and do another 8 weeks. You can add more weight, shorten your rest periods. I will be devising more intense kettlebell workouts in the future.

CHAPTER FIVE

Living the Healthy Lifestyle

Knowing how to maintain your target weight will help you avoid wasting all of your hard work once you've achieved it. When you reach the point where you have accomplished your weight loss goal, the knowledge you have gained in advance will be helpful. You obviously want to keep up your newly discovered healthy lifestyle and would not want to ruin the celebration you will want to have.

Never skip a meal: Keep in mind that your metabolism will interpret this as a sign that you are starving and start to store fat as a reserve. Make sure to continue eating your meals as you have been planning them. Furthermore, skipping a meal at one point during the day may result in overeating later on when you are simply too hungry.

Continue to eat a variety of foods: This will make it easier for you to continue getting all the vitamins and nutrients your body needs to stay healthy. It will keep your body healthy, give you energy, and safeguard your body by doing so. Whole grains, fruits, vegetables, and lean proteins are among the options you have. Keep up your workouts! Don't become complacent and stop working out right away.

If you received instruction from a personal trainer, you now know what kind of exercise is best for you and probably how to switch things up occasionally as well.

It's a good idea to switch up your routine occasionally to prevent boredom and keep your body on its toes. You will continue to stay in shape, feel strong and healthy, and you will further protect yourself from illnesses when you combine your cardio and strength training with a healthy diet.

Start with just 250 extra calories per day. Check your weight once a week. Most likely, you still have some additional weight to lose. If so, increase your calorie intake by another 250, then weigh yourself a week later.

When you weigh yourself at the end of the week, keep going through these steps until you see that your weight has stayed the same. If you've gained a little weight, reduce it by 100 calories at a time until it stabilizes and stays the same from week to week.

Continue consuming that water: Drink at least eight glasses of water daily to keep your body functioning properly. Drinking water improves digestion, gives you more energy, and aids in the natural detoxification of your body. You will also continue to be healthy and hydrated.

Continue to eat frequently: You have probably already figured out that eating five to six small meals a day is a good idea because it keeps your metabolism going and leaves you feeling satisfied.

It is crucial to keep doing this as well because, if this was a problem in the past, you don't want to fall into the trap of increasing your portion sizes once more. One day you'll find yourself right back where you started. You will at the very least put on a lot of the weight you worked so hard to lose back.

Keep the junk food outside: Why ruin your new healthy habits by reverting to your old behaviors and overindulging in junk food? You've learned how to satisfy all of your cravings with delicious, nutritious foods. Maintain a daily intake of fruits and vegetables of at least six to eight servings.

Take your vitamins each day. Do not stop taking your daily vitamin supplements. You can ensure that you get all the vitamins you need each day by doing this, which will also help you keep a healthy weight.

The Secrets of Staying Healthy

Everybody wants to live long and healthy lives; nobody wants to count on getting any severe diseases. There are ways to help protect ourselves that can help make our lives more full and healthy overall, even though we can't predict or prevent every situation.

You should prioritize early detection and prevention first. Most people dread getting their yearly physicals or even going to the dentist every six months for a cleaning. However, keeping these appointments and finding good doctors will help you stay healthy because they can spot things that you can't.

Knowing your family history is essential because your doctor can monitor your symptoms and perform routine testing if there is a history of cancer or heart disease in your family.

Respect the company you keep. Spend time with the people who are always there for you, such as your spouse, kids, extended family, friends, and coworkers. Enjoy your interactions with others and uphold wholesome friendships. You need these connections in order to feel fulfilled in life.

Sleep for eight hours. Despite the fact that many people find this one challenging given how busy our lives can become, it is actually crucial to living a happy and healthy life.

Find a skill you excel at. Everybody has moments when they should be doing something they really enjoy, and most of the time, these moments call for their best abilities. Typically, this also gives us a positive internal feeling and may even be calming and stress-relieving.

Don't ignore your stress; manage it instead! Everyone experiences some form of stress, and it's crucial that we manage it to prevent it from becoming overwhelming and taking over our lives.

You can actually become physically ill when you are plagued by worry and stress in a number of ways. Daily walks can help you relax and check that your schedule is not too full or that you are not letting other people's schedules control your day.

Obtain equilibrium in your life. Try not to let work consume you or attempt not to take on too many projects. Find a balance so you are still able to enjoy all the other things around you like your hobbies and your friends and family.

Even though times can be difficult financially, it is still crucial to make time for your family, whom you work so hard to protect and provide for.

The Advantages of Staying Healthy

The advantages of maintaining good health are endless. It's not just that you can fit into that new outfit and are content with the way you look. Your overall physical, mental, and social wellbeing are all impacted by your level of health.

Your Physical Health: Maintaining good physical health will benefit you in all respects. It not only enables you to participate in daily activities like walking, moving, and bending, but it also gives you the physical capacity to look after your dependent family members.

If you avoid diseases that were preventable and that would be very expensive, it may be financially advantageous.

Your Mental Health: If your mental health is poor, it will also have an impact on your physical health. Many people are unaware of the significance of their mental health to their general wellbeing. It can make you ill if you let yourself become overly stressed or if that stress takes control of your life.

Your risk of having a heart attack or stroke increases if you are under stress. You must find healthy ways to manage your stress, such as through exercise, meditation, or therapy. Avoid handling stress in unhealthy ways, such as by smoking, drinking, or eating unhealthful foods.

Disease Prevention: Maintaining overall health and staying healthy requires eating a healthy diet. Your health may be directly affected by the foods you choose to eat.

Phytochemicals are crucial for your health and may help ward off conditions like high blood pressure, certain types of cancer, diabetes, and heart disease. Only certain foods, including berries, spinach, olives, and kale, contain them. Consume a low-fat diet rich in whole grains, fruits, and vegetables to help safeguard your cardiovascular health.

Long Life: Maintaining a healthy lifestyle can play a significant role in your ability to live a long and active life. Even though you can't prevent all health issues and some of them are beyond your control, leading a healthy lifestyle can help you avoid many of the most serious ones.

Having a healthy lifestyle that includes managing your diet is crucial because chronic diseases like diabetes, heart disease, cancer, and stroke are the leading causes of death. Maintaining a healthy weight, how much you exercise, and how you handle stress in your life can all have a significant impact on preventing these diseases.

Maintaining a healthy lifestyle can also lift your spirits, increase your sense of worth, and sharpen your mind. You will be more physically fit, have more endurance, and be able to sleep better at night.

Improved digestion and lower blood pressure are two additional advantages of leading a healthy lifestyle. Maintaining good health can also help you reduce or completely get rid of back pain and problems, as well as enhance your balance and coordination, posture, and resting heart rate.

Everyone is aware of what to do now that they have learned how to change their lifestyle and lose weight. They read the information and realize they must act and exert effort, but the reality is that people rarely do. You will struggle to start down the path to a healthy life unless you have the self-control to fight the urge to eat unhealthy foods and the motivation to eat healthy foods.

If you don't take that first step, no amount of reading or affirming your ability to succeed will be of any use to you. Both the initial commitment and the ongoing commitment are extremely difficult to maintain. Most people give up quickly because they are dissatisfied with their outcomes. You will succeed in your mission if you can stay committed, maintain your motivation, and keep setting healthy eating and exercise goals for yourself. You just need to go out there and put in the necessary effort and work, regardless of your goals—whether they are to lose weight, build endurance, or improve as an athlete in a particular sport.

Over time, you'll not only mentally get used to your training schedule, but you'll also gain a lot of self-control, discipline, and confidence. You'll also naturally keep a positive outlook, which makes it simple to withstand temptation.

Each person must begin their journey somewhere. Instead of attempting to go all-out and try to sweat out 10 pounds on the treadmill over the course of a week, setting your goals gradually will be more beneficial. Starting the process slowly is important, so take a brisk walk to help your body adjust to the more strenuous runs you intend to do in the following weeks.

One error beginners make is going all out, which results in injury and prompts them to quickly decide that training is simply too painful and taxing.

As before, make a schedule and, if necessary, speak with a personal trainer about what might be best for you if making a schedule makes you uncomfortable. You don't need to make the procedure so challenging, in my opinion. If you want to lose weight, all you really need to do is set aside a brief period of time each day for exercise and monitor your diet.

Be confident and make progress toward your objectives. Being optimistic will help you achieve your goals. Maybe now is a good time to start making that plan and acting so you can get on the path to the super healthy lifestyle you deserve as the start of a new season draws near.